For years I have seen people exercise vigorously lifting heavy weights, running and walking with little to no results. Most people think that if they can just find more time to exercise the excess weight will just melt away. So they join gyms hire trainers or buy another piece of fad equipment that promises amazing results.

Then there are all the different diet products. Saturday and Sunday mornings as well as late night television will not let you sleep until you've heard about some new successful diet. The weight loss industry is giant and growing. There seems to be a multinational industrial supplement and diet complex developing.

For good reason were interested in our health. It's personal and it affects us daily and it affects our future. The goal of this book is to give you true and simple principles that will help you navigate past all the pop advice and clever marketing. The truth is that dieting should be simple, but it is not. We are targets of the health industry. You are being pulled in every direction by bad advice marketed as 'healthy'. Much of it is just the opposite of healthy. If it was possible to take profits out of the equation the advice would be clear, it would be simpler.

I will try to appeal to your sense of reason, not talk over your head with fitness and nutritions' higher criticism or confusing shop lingo. You will receive sound principles that are easy to remember. My goal is the clarity and simplicity that were all starving for. Therefore I make much use of memory devices to help you keep hold of the principles given.

Yes this book has handles. The advice herein should be easy to pick up, carry with you and share with others. Some who give diet advice treat it as water balloons. It's hard to keep and carry with you. Also it's awkward and you must be very careful with it. Those type diets are only good for one thing, throwing at others.

When you share this information with your friends, family or clients they won't run in fear screaming, but it can be easily grasped, welcomed and held.

But I Am Eating Healthy!

Why Popular Health Advice is Keeping You From Losing Weight

Chapter 1

How To Gain Weight

You say, 'I don't need help with this.' I know, don't be shocked that this chapter is included in the book. That's not the goal you're reaching for, but here's the problem. The same strategies some will give you to lose weight are the same strategies we use to help athletes and others gain weight. Yes much of the effort you've put in over the years could have been playing sabotage with your diet.

Just as a train goes in reverse before it goes forward, you need to back up in your thinking. If a person desires to gain weight no nutritionist or dietitian in his or her right mind is going to recommend eating in an unhealthy way to gain weight. They will always suggest healthy strategies in order to achieve weight gain.

Likely you've used many of these strategies in an effort to lose weight. Don't be ashamed, many people have. I've heard so many say, 'But I am eating healthy!' or they may say, 'You're not going to believe this, but I really don't eat a lot'. I know. I believe you.
But here's what you should know:

To gain weight:

1. Eat yogurt.
Many yogurts on the market are calorie dense foods. They advertise their tastiness because they have added enough sweeteners and artificial ingredients that it's not really like yogurt anymore. Even if it is yogurt, its dairy

fat. Natural fats are good for your body, of course they are. But this is still a fast and easy way to add dense calories to your diet. Albeit healthy calories.

2. Put fruit in the yogurt.
Fruit adds taste and flavor. We shouldn't neglect the vitamins and minerals present in fruit. Once again, it's an easy and healthy way to add calories.

3. Drink milk.
Later we will discuss the benefits of milk and it's uptake in the muscles. Like yogurt it's dense dairy fat and calories. Milk helps young animals and babies gain weight to be healthy and grow. But if you're finished growing you may only get one of the main benefits of milk, weight gain.

4. Drink high fat or chocolate milk. So many studies
laud the benefits of chocolate. Exercise magazines may recommend it as a good post workout recovery. The artificial sugars, colors, and stabilizers therein all will help in our efforts to gain weight.

5. Eat multigrain Bagels.
It is healthy grains right? Not necessarily. But even so, eaten at the right times we can contribute to your healthy weight gain.

6. Use peanut butter on the bagels.
Fat and flavor and dense calories are naturally included. Peanut butter doesn't have to be unhealthy to contribute to weight gain

7. Eat meal replacement bars or energy bars.
This is a good and quick way to get dense carbohydrates. Since their easily consumed and travel well, you can add calories anywhere.

8. Don't replace the meals.
Fruit smoothies and meal replacement bars consumed at the proper times will not interrupt appetite at meal time allowing you to eat more.

9. Eat 5-6 meals daily.
Again we have to add calories. If you tried to eat everything in one setting it would be impossible. So spread your increased calories throughout the day. This way it will be easier to eat more.

10. Use butter & olive oil in food preparation.
Butter and Olive oil is very good in food preparation. I recommend them over chemical spreads and sprays. Using them correctly will make it possible to use more of them and as a result get more calories.

Most of the above strategies are healthy. So don't go out and buy other items thinking you are avoiding some list of bad foods. The repetitive point is adding calories, especially in the areas of fats and carbohydrates, leads to weight gain. This is healthy weight gain, which many people unknowingly practice. Of course there are many unhealthy ways to gain weight. Being aware of the healthy strategies of weight gain gives you better decision making abilities.

Web MD and others reported on the negative effects of sugars in the diet. But is sugar really the problem or artificial sugars? You be the judge.

In San Antonio, Texas 5000 people were followed over a period of 7 years. Those who drank diet sodas gained more weight over time than those drinking regular sodas. What does this tell you about diet drinks? Have you noticed the people in the real world that drink the diet drinks? They're not like the skinny well shaped models on the commercials.

Artificial sugars actually increase your appetite! Yes their zero calories but they make you consume more. Why would any diet product want you to consume more? The study compared real sugar to artificial sugars. Notice I used the adjective 'real'. If you've ever been to South America or the Caribbean you will notice sugar cane is a plant, it's a vegetable. It's one of the beneficial plants. Of course you can have too much of anything. But we all have to quit being afraid of real sugar. If you want to fear, be afraid of chemically processed artificial sugars. They have been shown to make people fatter than the zero calorie alternatives. The same results in weight gain were shown in humans and rats that were studied.

So how can you gain weight? First follow temporary diets, drink diet sodas, use artificial sweeteners, and sadly buy diet products. Now here's the rub where you will get into trouble listening to pop advice. Notice the take away given by a popular web site.

"Because both of these studies were observational, it is impossible to say if the diet sodas played a direct role in the weight gain." (Web MD)

No matter what the negative results are the answer is always we need more studies. Look at your family and friends. The studies went one way in humans and rats. The subjects gained weight even with zero calorie alternatives. Even more weight with the zero calorie sweeteners than the natural in most cases. Let them experiment with the chemical artificial sugars but you use plant based minimally processed sugar. Over a hundred years your grandparents and parents used table sugar, even the white variety. But your generation, the one given the pink, yellow, and blue sugars became the balloons.

Let the giant companies defend their products. You defend your family. Our bodies know well how to deal with carbs, protein, fats, vitamins, minerals & water. Sugar is a (CHO) carbohydrate. It's one of the necessary nutrients. Chemical substances in food have to be filtered, dispose of or assimilated. Can you feel satiety, or get a feeling of fullness from chemicals as you do when you eat natural food? Is that what you want? Is that what your body wants or needs? Of course not. Experts, especially those not in the field of weight loss, do not have a monopoly on common sense.

Chapter 2

Avoid Diet Foods

Recently Weight Watchers changed its point system to emphasize quality calories over quantity of calories. Fruits and Vegetable are now zero points. Now you can have unlimited quantities of these with their system. Proteins and fibers have lower point values while fats have higher point value. Points control not only quantity but also quality now.

Now it's very close to the advice I give. They deserve much credit for this change. But many of these programs have stood behind processed food companies and endorsed their products.

Food companies have little love for you personally. The convenience of processed foods is what get us in trouble. They're addictive; they're big on flavor. That flavor comes from bad salts, bad sugars, and bad fats. I framed these words with the adjective 'bad'. Because these three items also come in 'good' varieties. Once again, to put them in the same category with good salts, sugars, and fats would be a travesty.

There are real sugar then fake sugars, good salts and fats then bad salts and fats. Many diet foods do not differentiate but your body will. You cannot live without sugar, salt or fat. In fact it's dangerous to try. And the good stuff isn't usually found in processed or diet foods. Then there's the zero calorie craze. Every fitness trainer in their study guides and training will hear calories in calories out. So they relay that thinking you. Calories count, but all calories aren't created equal. The calories in calories out advice push and drive people to zero calorie products. This is not the best strategy. Here's why.

This is an example why calories aren't the whole picture.

- Zero calorie artificial sweeteners can actually increase appetite!
- Refined calories are superglue for fat since they provide little to no insulin reducing agents like nutrients or fiber. So the same amounts of refined calories have a higher fat storage effect.
- High glycemic calories speeds fat storage.
- Timing of calories influence metabolic use or storage. At high metabolic times, calories burn faster.

This Calories in Calories out formula can be misleading. There are a couple of other circumstances that deflate the hype.

1. Water has no calories but if you drink three glasses you gain one pound. One pound of weight with no calories involved.

2. It takes calories to digest food. If you eat 100 calories of fat it takes about 3 calories to assimilate it. Some proteins

and fibers can use up to 15% or more of the calories in the breakdown. So a 500 calorie meal can result in a lesser caloric intake.

3. Sugar spikes from lots of calories eaten at one setting make extra sugar in the bloodstream. The extra is then stored away as fat. So 2000 calories throughout the day is better than a single 2000 calorie meal.

If only companies would quit marketing refined, artificial and processed foods! Can we really count on companies to leave quickly degradable good nutrients that reduce shelf life in foods? Not if doing this will lower their profits.

Some of the most popular of diets restrict essential nutrients. For instance some diets tell you to not eat fruit. Others say not to eat potatoes. What! Fruits can be considered diet pills. They have essential acids in proper balance, fiber as well as micronutrients and phytonutrients that science still cannot explain all of the benefits.

Whenever we restrict proper nutrition our bodies are going to crave to make it up. We're designed to pull nutrients from foods. So your body has a choice when you diet. Get nutrients when and while you can or do without them. Going too long without proper nutrition may

well
make us stock up when we can.

It's like being in the southern U.S. when it snows. Whether you need it or not people stock up on staples out of fear of doing without. Diets may well put our bodies in a snow scare or gas crisis. Top off your tank now because something is wrong with the supply chain.

So can you ever go on a diet? Well the Greek word for diet means 'way of life'. Changing your way of life is what you must do. Here are some principles about dieting that will help.

· Diets should be easy to remember & follow. What's the point if you need a technical writing degree or become a mathematician to follow a certain diet?
· Diets should be inexpensive or free.
· The best foods to eat are inexpensive. And of course the best thing to drink is free. Exactly what are they selling you?
· You should see results every two weeks. (inches, energy, appetite or lbs.) Likely you won't be able to eat enough. Yeah, the good foods are calorie sparse but nutrient dense. But you must eat to see results you want.
· Also they should allow for foods you actually like to eat. (Changes you can live with) who wants to live in a world without dessert?
There's a place and time for your favorite foods. If they are not desserts, they may need to be treated like desserts. Not eaten daily, and after the good stuff.

· They should include recommended daily allowances of whole grains + vegetables. If you are told not to eat essential nutrients in their natural forms or cause a nutritional deficit by eliminating an entire
food group that diet isn't long term or reasonable.
· Skipping meals is not a long term beneficial strategy. Fasting can be beneficial, especially if you're trying to break a negative food cycle. But this can lead to so many problems. Remember how the weight came? Slowly over time. Trying to slice off a pound of flesh overnight is dangerous.
· Lastly you should have a dated goal. The entire human existence is a story of hope, milestones and goals. Monitor your progress. But remember progress should be wholistic. Were you successful in your timing of meals? For instance, adding water to your meals, increasing vegetables, your energy, your knowledge of foods and their content. All of this is progress along with pounds inches and strength.

Too many people are trying to sell us on quick weight loss & uncontrolled eating without exercise. Or exercise without dieting. Foods marketed diet or healthy are in some cases worse than their cheaper or free counterparts. Then ergogenic aids and weight loss supplements are an expensive way to get nutrients you can get better from readily available foods. Frankly the food media will help you do the opposite of exactly what you're trying to accomplish. Eat clean, real, food in the right portions. But how can you know exactly what that is? Keep reading.

Chapter 3

Likely You Need To Eat More

Yes, you likely need to eat more. Overweight people are always telling their closest friends and relatives that they really aren't eating a lot of food. Some never really voice the words because of the imagined looks of disbelief. Even moderately overweight people may be under eating. So let me get this out of the way. Eat unlimited fruits and vegetables. Unlimited, without limits. Let me illustrate how this works by using iodine.

After the Japan and other nuclear accidents people were advised to take iodine. This was because there was radioactive iodine in the environment. Taking good clean iodine fills the iodine stores or nutritional needs so you don't take in radioactive iodine.

Don't fear eating lots of good nutrient rich fruits and vegetables. Get everything you need from these first. There's no reason to be hungry, you can eat unlimited fruits and vegetables. It's hard to over eat on these.

So what about controlling portions? Control the less healthy foods just like you control your alcohol intake. So how can you do this? Instead of trying to eat 5 or 6 meals a day, take an hour and plan 6 good meals of 6 good options. So on the days you don't know what to eat, you have 6 options to draw from. Later we will discuss how to set the recommended amounts of the options. Here's a sample outline below.

6 Meal Plan

You should take a minute and create a meal plan. You need a total of six different meals. 2 breakfast, 2 lunches, 2 dinners & 2 snacks

Breakfast (small) where? home/restaurant
-protein source_____
-whole grain_____
-fruits_____
-vegetables_____

SNACK (fruit or veggie)_____

Lunch where? home/restaurant
-protein source_____
-whole grain_____
-fruits_____
-vegetables_____

SNACK (fruit or veggie)_____

Dinner (small) where? home/restaurant
-protein source_____
-whole grain_____
-fruits_____
-vegetables_____

Eat this way 5 days a week. Ideally you want more fruits & veggies
than any thing else.

Breakfast (small) where? home/restaurant
-protein source_____
-whole grain_____
-fruits_____
-vegetables_____

SNACK (fruit or veggie)_____

Lunch where? home/restaurant
-protein source_____
-whole grain_____
-fruits_____
-vegetables_____

SNACK (fruit or veggie)_____

Dinner (small) where? home/restaurant
-protein source_____
-whole grain_____
-fruits_____
-vegetables_____

If you eat out, choose unprocessed lean meats, whole grains, and add every vegetable possible. Avoid if possible fried & breaded foods. All the restaurants have 1 to 2 good choices. They may be more expensive in the smaller restaurants but you should spend the money and get the good stuff.

How can you know how much of what to eat? Well Eat with Your Hands. Not really using your hands to eat but use the memory method described in chapter 9 of this book. This Method will help you remember and to get your Recommended Daily Intake of the proper foods.

How Much Protein Do You Need?

It's not too hard to calculate your protein intake needs. There's a couple of simple ways that will apply to most people. But protein is virtually useless in burning fat without utilizing carbs and fat. Never go all protein! Your body needs the other nutrients also. So really what is needed is knowledge of the daily intake of all three carbs, protein and fat plus the right water intake to perform at your best.

Are you better with having a number to follow? There's easy ways for that also. .

Protein= Half your body weight (grams)
Carbs = Body weight+half body weight
Fat. = 10% body weight (chose low fat)
Water = Half your body weight (oz.)

Most people get too many bad carbs and not enough good ones. It's the same with fats. Contrary to popular opinion excess protein can also become fat and you need more carbs than protein. Good carbs, clean carbs. There's a difference between the good and bad of course. And some are just plain ugly.

So sounds like you're going to be eating a lot of food right? Yes lots of food but not calorie dense foods. For instance, to eat what the body considers real food takes large amounts to sustain your daily requirements. (Nearly 6 apples for one snickers bar [537 Cal]) Can you eat 6 apples in the same time it takes to eat one Snickers bar?

Calories are important but again, all calories are not created equal. Good clean calories burn better. Most people will burn 1200 calories a day just lying in bed.

-Imagine if you were on a 1200-1500 calorie intake along with your regular daily routine.

-Imagine adding 500 calories a week in cardio or muscle training. (2 hours treadmill walk 1.5 hour dancing or 45 min fitness class)

Trying to get 1500 calories of good food is going to require some eating. At a restaurant this can be just one meal because they include so many of the worse calories. In any case you are burning calories every waking hour. That's why your body's warm to the touch. That's also why the dead are cold. At this point many still can't imagine trying to eat more. As you keep reading you'll get more tools to tailor your eating.

Forget about losing weight for now, but make a strong determination not to gain. (Trying not to gain actually often facilitates loss of weight) Here's the overriding principle you should work with at this point. It's easier to keep weight off than to take it off.

Chapter 4 Breakfast,

Not The Most Important Meal of The Day.

You may have heard so many people say, 'Eat a big breakfast. It's the most important meal of the day.' Or Breakfast like a King, lunch like a Prince and dinner like a Pauper. This is a big widespread and misleading myth.

Eat a big breakfast to get your metabolism going. Be less hungry throughout the day. (Bogus!) The idea is that you will eat in the form of a right triangle. Biggest meal to the smallest. Is that really how anyone eats? Is it how you eat? No!

Most people eat in a straight line averaging 800-1500 calories each meal. (Including beverages) In fact, a new study suggests that eating a big breakfast just adds calories, does not contribute to weight loss or increased metabolism.

So what can we say about the former pop advice that encourages loading at breakfast? The Emperor is finally getting a mirror. The Big Breakfast Lobby & Most Important meal people are beginning to see their logic is naked and fat.

Well you're asking, 'How should I eat throughout the day?' You've heard of the Food Pyramid & My Pyramid. They're made to make eating simple, but I doubt anyone really remembers their contents except nutritionist. Here's a new and easier one.

Pyramid Eating. Yes another Pyramid but this world wonder is memorable.

· Breakfast small

It's the bottom corner of the pyramid. You only need enough fuel to get you to lunch. Too much is extra weight. Unless you are a lumberjack using hand tools, you only need a few calories at this time. Remember you only have 2-3 hours to your next meal.

· Lunch tops the Pyramid

Here is your most active part of the day, fuel it. You have 4-8 hours till dinner. Eat now and smaller later. The best point here is that you usually have better self-control at this time. Also lunch menus are cheaper! Its been noted that those who take their lunch with them usually make better choices. It's the best time to really eat.

· Dinner at the bottom

The bottom corner of the Pyramid that is. Your next event is sleep. Here you don't need a lot of energy. In fact you don't want a lot of food or energy if you ate well at lunch. Try to eat 3-4 hours before bed.

Ideally you will snack after breakfast and lunch. This way of eating gives you fuel when you need it not when you don't. Every morning you should endeavor to start a metabolic fire. What do I mean?

Have you ever tried to start a fire with a large block of wood? You need an accelerant or kindling right? Trying to start your metabolism moving with a large meal is insane! You may just bog down the whole process.

First, start your fire with water. In the body water helps everything move and work. Water is a metabolic accelerant. Never let anyone convince you water is not important with diet or weight loss.Water is important to everything including weight loss. In fact calories are measured in terms of water temperature.

Next, use a small amount of fuel to get things hot. 300 calories or less then wait two to three hours before eating again.

Later at lunch put some wood on the fire. Get it hot get warm!

Here are some sample breakfast meals.
What to eat? (AM)
- 1 Egg white on whole wheat toast
- A Banana and apple
- 2/3 cup of whole grain cereal
- Yogurt w/fruit
- Apple with peanut butter

- 1 egg & veggie omelet w/salsa
- (Spinach, mushroom, tomato, etc.)
- Energy bar (clean, low cal, low sugar)
- 2 oatmeal cookies (not daily)

Do not eat the whole list. This is a small sample of the variety you can have to get the fire going.

A University of Connecticut study compared men who ate a bagel and yogurt to men who consumed one egg with toast for breakfast. These men ate the same caloric content but the protein rich egg actually reduced feelings of hunger throughout the day. Also the Egg Men felt more energetic. (Health Monitor 6/10)

One reason people have gotten used to eating a large generous breakfast is advertising. Yes, the Origins of Obesity is an evolutionary story. In the book, 'In Defense of Food' it was reported that Charles Darwin indirectly influenced our eating habits. What does Charles Darwin have to do with eating habits? In the 1920s most rural peoples ate only toast and coffee for breakfast. In an effort to sell more livestock, Farmers hired a Marketing Professional. The son of famed Evolutionist Charles Darwin. He conducted a survey of a few Doctors. Simply, "would you prefer people eat a large hearty breakfast or a small one?" .....hence more eggs, pork, milk, etc were sold.

Another Obesity Research study suggested portion control works better for weight loss than exercise, consuming less fat, and increasing fruits & veggies. (J Wiesenberger RD (pm6/10)) What's the point?

Controlling portions at the right times can be a very effective strategy. Most fitness trainers will tell you, 'abs are made in the kitchen not the gym.' Diet for weight loss, exercise to keep it off.

Ever heard of the Cup&Saucer Meal Plan discussed in Chapter 10? This will help you follow all these recommendations in an easy to remember format. Yes the Cup and Saucer Meal plan has handles.

Chapter 5

You're About to Save a Lot of Money

Where is your money going anyway? The expensive products are producing little in results. The advertising says they're made from 'something' natural or you get the same benefits as many times 'something' natural. This is the bottled water scam all over again.

Companies sell us packaged products that have the same benefits as water in the way of calories, same color, just as clean and refreshing with the same convenience but at 100 times the price.

As we must retrain ourselves to drink water, we must also retrain ourselves to eat fruits and vegetables. Vegetables and fruits are cheap, convenient, and fruits come with its own convenient biodegradable packaging.

Much of our time is wasted on the diet products and diets. The same goes with the time spent in the gym doing unproductive & unsafe routines. At the end of the book we will cover how to get the most out of your workouts. But for now we'll focus on how the most beneficial diets or ways of eating are actually very inexpensive. Notice this statistic.

Plate Size

In 60s & 70s standard dinner plate size increased from 9" to 11" in diameter. This increased size holds 50% more food. Today the standard European plates are still 9". (On Fitness Mag 12/10)

One reason we are bigger because our portions are bigger. We've been taught to eat a big breakfast. Why? We do not need that much energy to sustain us to lunch. Most peoples intervals between breakfast and lunch is 2 to 3 hours. A smaller cheaper breakfast is in order.

Small portions early are satisfying. In two hours if you get hungry eat small again. In fact this would be an excellent time to remember to drink water or eat fruit. Meats tend to be expensive, plus the breakfast meats are horrible for your health. Processed sausage, fried chicken, and salty varieties of other meats are among these.

If you can handle it, becoming an AM/PM vegetarian can be a beneficial health strategy. Only eating meats during lunch. But beware; many vegetarians are unhealthy because of relying on refined breads and starches. They should endeavor to put the vegetable back in vegetarian.

Personally I usually refrain from meat at breakfast and most dinners. I wouldn't totally give up on meat because it's still a good source of necessary nutrients and complete proteins. Still vegetarian diets have lots of benefits. We will cover some of these benefits since vegetables definitely need to make a comeback in the whole worlds eating habits. Think about these simple benefits.

○ You can eat a lot of food! As long as it's not processed, fruits and veggies are low calorie and high in water. They make you feel fuller with less.

○ Their Multi-Vitamins with flavor. There are substrates in natural foods that science has no idea how they work or how they benefit us. Among these are phytochemicals and phytonutrients.

○ You claim the high moral ground. Cows and chickens smile as you walk by. And every time you order a salad somewhere deep in the ocean a dolphin sees a rainbow.

○ Vegetables are cheap. This leaves more money for the new wardrobe you'll need.

So in what other ways will you save money? Small, simple breakfasts can be easily prepared and eaten quickly at home saving you the cost of drive thrus and the impulse spending that comes with them. Then a smaller portion at dinner is in order. Why continue on the large dinner plates. Take your eating back to the 60s and 70s when America used smaller plates. There's good reasons to reduce our plate size like the fact that smaller portions are less expensive.

We need to reinstate what some called a diet myth. So called Myth, 'Calories consumed at night are worse than at other times of day.' This is misleading. It would fit better under truth.

Here's why. Those who view this as a myth feel that no matter how or when you consume calories, an equal amount of calories equal an equal amount of weight. 3500 calories equals a pound fair and simple.

But are all types of calories equal? Is 3500 calories in hamburgers the same metabolically as 3500 calories in greens? No! Are all foods metabolized equally? No! Digested equally? No! Does metabolism act at a constant rate? No! Consider this.

Metabolic Economics.

All body functions slow at night. If you go to bed with a calorie deficit your body will breakdown muscle and fat to fill the glycogen stores in the liver and muscles. Going to bed with a calorie surplus after energy stores are full will lead to fat storage.

During the day glycogen stores are constantly being depleted and replaced. Energy is being used and metabolic rates are higher. It takes about 4 hours to refill energy stores. Within 1 hour food is being converted to energy. This is why bodybuilders eat within an hour after exercise. During sleep there's less conversion and more storage.

Sports Nutritionists call this Carb Timing. Athletes are not to eat a big meal within an hour before activity. There's no time to convert the energy and they just become sluggish.

In addition foods use a range of caloric energy in digestion. They actually burn calories while you consume them. A 100 calorie food could only result in 97 calories of value because 3 calories were used to breakdown the food.

The same calories can be stored and used very differently based on type and timing. I promised not to use complicated terminology so here's a simple illustration.

Too Much Inventory at night is just too much. What happens to the stock delivered to a grocery store at night? First the shelves are filled, the overstock it stored. There's not much traffic at night and product hardly moves.

Our bodies are similar; at night we store 1 to 3 hours of energy in our muscles and liver about 100-300 calories depending on our body. Anything over our energy stores is put into our fat storage. Most people get 3-5 deliveries a day. In the morning and at night we don't need a lot of product on our shelves. Do not stock up at night unless you want to gain weight.

Carb Timing is eating the right carbs before competition or one hour after workouts increases performance and spikes insulin in order to accelerate muscle repair. (Right, there are times you should spike insulin) Carb timing should be practiced at low RMR times also. Or when your metabolism is slowed and energy production is minimized.

Night time would be a good time to watch intake amounts. Not just Carb timing but calorie timing should be considered. Like an airplane just carry enough fuel till your next destination. At night your next destination is sleep. The body is on autopilot at night and really don't need a lot of energy at this time. Too much fuel just makes you too heavy.

Self-Test: Eat a big meal and go to bed. Wake up hungry. Where did the food go? Eat a very small portion before bed. No hunger in the morning? Where did the body get the energy? Why are you not hungry?

Your body has energy stored. If it needs more while you sleep, it will find it in fat storage. Smaller dinners prevent unused energy in the bloodstream at night. Unused latent energy is called fat.

Another way to save money is quit buying diet pills and drinks. Quit using meal replacement smoothies and bars. Overall they're worthless. Actually their expensive, but their value does not justify the price. Just save your money.

Chapter 6

Salt, Sugar, and Fat gets a Bad R.A.P.

Needless to say most Americans are getting too much salt, sugar and fat. But of course there are the good and bad varieties of each.

Salt, sugar and fats are all essential to a healthy life. Focusing on Salt, Sugar and Fat deflects attention from the guys that really deserve a bad (R.A.P.) Refined, Artificial and Processed foods. Salt, sugar and fat are Real food, natural food and fine in the right types and amounts. If we prefer real food we will naturally reduce the bad varieties while increasing the good varieties.

Are refined artificial and processed foods really that bad?

`During World War II Denmark stopped refining flour, an action which was not accompanied by any other marked changes in living habits. Later it was found that the death rate had dropped and that there had been a marked decline in cancer, heart disease, diabetes, kidney trouble, and high blood pressure.' (Mental And Elemental Nutrients, Carl C. Pfeiffer, Ph.D., M.D. p.72)

Laboratory animals cannot live for more than a few weeks on white bread, yet most of us like eating this denatured and impoverished food.' (Rex Newnham, Odyssey, Dec/Jan 1983/4, p.14)

Should you totally give up refined artificial and processed foods? Well should you totally give up ice cream and cake? No, I would never suggest that. Just as ice cream and cake needs to be a minimum part of our overall diet refined, artificial, and processed foods cannot and should not be a main food source. They are desserts in disguise!

One item you may have been trying to cut back on is salt. You may actually need MORE salt than less. Really, is there anyone in the country that needs more salt? How do you know if you're not getting enough salt? Think of how you prepare food. Are you adding more than two teaspoons of salt daily? What about sugar? Are you adding lots of sugar? It's not us it's them. Food manufacturers are making the big additions not us.

I expect those who read this book not to rely heavily on processed manufactured foods. So how will you get your salt? If you're eating fresh, clean, lean, and green you could be at risk for a salt deficiency.

In the 80's the increase in Chronic Fatigue was said to be mainly due to people cutting too much salt from their diet. Also low salt increases insulin resistance. Meaning it prevents you from turning food into energy or burning fat. So salt is a necessary nutrient. Times when you may need more salt is during hot weather and exercise periods.

For example it is recommended to add salt to your water if you are experiencing muscle twitches during exercise. Also add salt to your water if you lose more than a pound of sweat during exercise. Again if you're consuming lots of processed foods, be careful about ever adding more salt to your diet. They've done it for you. And it's not the good variety; likely it's sodium nitrates.

Sugar as you know has also been demonized so much that now there are so many alternatives to sugar. I really don't want this book to become a sort of defense of sugar. But just as the low to no carb craze demonized bread, real sugar has suffered the same fate. All breads good and bad suffered at that time.

Real sugar needs to be separated from the artificial and chosen over processed varieties. Sugar is your bodies' main source of energy (CHO). Carbs are sugar. Of all chemicals we consume, our bodies knows well how to use sugar. Some have decided to substitute sugar with sweet agave nectar. Ounce per ounce it's the same caloric and glycemic value as sugar. Some varieties have even more calories than sugar. It's a natural alternative but it's also more expensive!

If you've ever been in the fields of Hawaii or the Loma's of the Dominican Republic or the cost of Louisiana you've seen or even bitten into pure sugar cane. It grows naturally. It's a sweet stick. Sugar also helps you feel full strengthening your willpower.

That's why I suggest to anyone who's trying to break free from a soda addiction to switch to natural sugar sodas instead of diet sodas. Like Mexican Coke. It's still made with real sugar. Real sugar drinks are less toxic, less addictive, more filling and less sweet. Daily in the media you will hear sugar being slandered. It's setup as a monster to be feared. If you want fear, fear the chemical sweeteners. And beware of 'made from', or 'zero calorie' sweeteners.

Even celery and lettuce isn't a zero calorie food. Zero calorie means water or not food. Is there a place for artificial sugars other than the trash can? I'm not a fan of them at all, but I have to be fair. Artificial sugars are cheaper. Some varieties are not easily metabolized and claim to go right through you, but so can a bullet. Will they really go through your liver and kidneys with no biological response? Companies can lower the prices of products using these sweeteners. They're usually sweeter. You can use less to get similar or more taste.

They're patriotic also. America grows a lot of corn that can be converted into sugar. Other countries cannot control the price of a staple America produces so abundantly.

Then diabetics are told these are better alternatives for controlling their sugar cravings. Health wise, diabetics may do better just staying away from all processed sugars. And its lack of metabolism (which they claim) doesn't mean there's no effect on the body the liver and triglycerides. When it comes to nutrition and weight loss, simple minimally processed plant based ground sugar is the overall better choice.

What about coffee should you drink It? Today it's bad, tomorrow it's good it seems. Saying coffee is bad is a hard sell. And every article I read seems to extol its greatness. It's made mostly of water and beans. The caffeine and oral hygiene may be of issue but the benefits are well also defined. I would be more concerned of what is added to the coffee. In any case, it's always a good idea to alternate every cup with a cup of water.

Some Asian and French coffees add chicory, which is a probiotic. In fact it's the main probiotic in some supplements. When it comes to the caffeine, many sports drinks add caffeine to boost energy. Also it's the top weight loss supplement. But isn't caffeine a diuretic? This story has been told before. Diuretics make you void water or urinate more. It is as much as a diuretic as water. It takes nearly 200-300 milligrams before a noticeable difference takes place. Most cups of coffee have about 20 milligrams of caffeine. So about 20 to 30 cups will make you have to run to the restroom more. But so will 20-30 cups of water. Then if you add carbohydrates like cream and sugar to coffee, it will slow down the need to empty the bladder.

(Reference this here)
http://www.health.harvard.edu/press_releases/coffee_he
alth_risk.htm

http://men.webmd.com/features/coffee-new-health-food

Lastly, when it comes to fat, I think the word has been out for a time that vegetables, nuts and fruits have good fats.

What about the dairy products? Well if you're going to choose, choose natural dairy products over artificial chemicals ones, by now you should know which is better. Of course it's the real food. Butter over margarine, milk over milk like products, cheese over cheese food. Can anyone really beat the taste of real dairy anyway? This one should be easy.

There's a surprising fact about natural milk proteins that should mentioned at this time. The protein uptake for muscle recovery is nearly 97%. This is better or equal to the synthetic or ergogenic aids used by some to build muscle. There's no need for protein supplements if you can drink milk. It is tops when it comes to muscle repair and regrowth. I usually tell individuals trying to lose weight to go for lower fat milk because fat should be a smaller part of a healthy diet. It's an important part although. The body uses acids from fats to breakdown fat in the body.

So going totally fat free can hinder weight loss. How can you tell if it's a good fat? Can you take it from its natural form to the dinner plate all at home? I mean if you had a cow, goat or presses for oils. Basically, is it simply made or do you have no earthly idea what it is or how it's made.

For instance what is canola oil? Ever ate a canola? How do you make corn oil? What vegetables are in vegetable oil? These names are as misleading as baby oil. Just use what you know.

Chapter 7

So You're Hungry, Now What?

You've tried to eat right. Watch your calories. Minimized all sugars, dairy & alcohol. But cravings are driving your appetite like a Mack truck. Now what? Give in, but just a little. Here's how.

· First slow it with water, even the fastest vehicles meets resistance in water.

· Next, offer a Piece Treaty. A piece of a healthy treat. Fruits and
vegetables have appeased kings and stopped many wars between savages.

· Lastly, give a little. There's a reason you have a craving, let it
have its voice. But just a little, remember cravings can have their
say but not their way.

The idea that 'Water will curb your appetite' is actually helpful. Some dismiss this advice as myth. It is tricky because appetite and hunger is different. Water can expand your stomach. It also can speed nutrient delivery to the bloodstream, which curbs hunger. But a person who ate a big meal can still have an appetite without being hungry. So appetite can be a unicorn. It can be a mental thing not really related to what you really need or even a learned behavior. 'We always eat this at this time.' Smell can also trigger it as well as nutritional deficiencies. In fact appetite is so complicated it would be hard for anyone to say they have full knowledge of it.

Here's the big question though. Do you really have an appetite? Don't answer so quickly. When thirst sets in you are already close to dehydration. Sometimes the thing you need the most when you have an 'appetite' is water.

Water plays a big part in perceived satisfaction. Different foods have Satiety Levels or satisfaction levels. (Some websites have a satiety index you can download for reference) The Satiety levels have much to do with how much water content is in the food. Water is one of the main factors in this index along with fiber. As illustrated in the satiety index, water is the first defense for cravings.

So here's the proven research:

-Drink water first
-Go for the good stuff next. Fresh, lean, clean, or green food in small amounts. These are the foods with higher satiety. But they have the added benefits of a few other nutrients that help, protein, fiber and sugar. When these enter the bloodstream they send signals to the brain that says, 'we're eating'.
-Wait 15-30 minutes. Those signals are slow. Give them a little time.
-Give in to the craving, just a little. Cravings could signal there's a nutritional deficit present, so listen to your body. Your body is making a suggestion not a decision.

Remember don't sweat it our appetite keeps us alive. It is how we know were alive. Like anything a new way of eating takes a while to get used to. Use your 6 Meal Plan to preempt any cravings that may occur. Also the Cup and Saucer meal plan discussed in Chapter 10 should counter any cravings. Remember that meal plan will give you unlimited fruits and vegetables.

Chapter 8

Make Your Own Diet Pills

Why buy diet pills when you can just make your own diet pills. I'm not suggesting you turn your kitchen into a crack house or health lab. Some of the most popular diet pills on the market can be replaced. How? By natural and common foods, vitamins or substrates.

B12 -popular doctors' weight loss shots are nothing more than a vitamin injection. This increases your energy so you're able to do more throughout the day and burn more calories as a result. B12 can be purchased for little or nothing at most vitamin stores. Even better it's found in common lean meats.

Fiber -one weight loss pill says it helps cut the calories in the food you eat. So does fiber! It helps prevent insulin spikes so excess blood sugar isn't converted to fat. Plus it gives a feeling of satiety. Yes it makes you feel full.

Caffeine -if a pill says it speeds your metabolism likely the first ingredient is caffeine. Many of the other ingredients that are included in supplements have little effect or are without scientific merit as of yet.

Ketones -HGC is all the rave now. Pregnant mothers' bodies use this chemical to breakdown fat. Trace amounts can be found in the urine of a pregnant woman. Ketones also breakdown fat. You get them by switching your body from sugar fueled to producing ketones. How?, the exact same way the HGC priest encourage. Severely reduce your caloric intake to a modified fast. As result your body has to use its fat stores for energy. When you switch to fat fueled you're not hungry because your body is eating. It's eating stored fat. The Adkins Diet is mainly based on the work of ketones. It worked by making a nutritional deficit in the way of carbohydrates.

Your physician should carefully monitor any modified fast. Although fasting has been practiced for centuries, there are inherent risks. The point is that all of these methods work. You can get them the expensive way or the free way.

By the way, every fruit and every vegetable is a diet pill. They give you energy; they have fiber, short term energy and long term energy. Since they are low calorie but high in satiety they curb your appetite. Unlike the diet drinks that may actually increase appetite. Then there's the nutrient balance, which we still don't fully understand is prefixed in these natural diet pills to give you maximum nutrient delivery. The benefit of a good diet is that you get all of these benefits naturally and they're less expensive.

In order to continue to shed pounds it may be healthful to consider the relationship of four foods. Fiber, Fruit, Fish & Fat.

Sounds like a Dr. Seuss book right? Well if it was, it would be about a fat cat that lowered his stats. I grouped them this way to make them easy to remember. By now you should have noticed a lot of memory devices in this book. R.A.P. Refined Artificial Processed, Cup & Saucer, Pyramid Eating, Eat with Your Hands, and others. So what about this fab four? Fiber, Fruit, Fish & Fat.

Increasing fiber, fruit, and fish oil can have a profound effect on heart health and reduce fat retention. Of course if we increase one area we should balance it with a decrease of the bad fatty oils and fatty meats. Now here's an anecdotal situation I personally experienced. I took a blood test for health insurance that revealed my cholesterol to be 205. So I decided to diet to lower my numbers. Within 3 weeks I took another blood test. My cholesterol was 165. What did I do? For the last week before the test, I consumed little to no animal products, and increased my fiber, which acts like a sponge for cholesterol.

As I said this is anecdotal, but it's a real example of the benefits of this way of eating. I recommend this type of eating for any of my clients that have photos or a special event coming in the near future. This way of eating has been labeled the DASH diet. Dietary Approaches to Suppress Hypertension. I call it the Photo Shoot Diet. It's a good lifestyle for almost everyone. Since it's very restrictive I don't think its long term for most people.

Portion control of course is the absolute fastest way to lose weight. Portion control isn't always the best though. Remember the weight came slow, and it should leave slowly for it to be long term. But portion control is a working method and should play a part of every diet.

Ever seen the pictures of skinny African Elephants? Yes skinny elephants exist. Elephants and Hippos are vegetarians. Food breaks downs in their systems similar to ours. They're also mammals. But most are big and fatty. Mainly for two reasons, genetics and portions. So what account for the skinny elephants? In some areas there isn't enough food. They're starving these elephants portions are reduced. Elephants prove being vegetarian doesn't mean being small. But it still can be a healthy lifestyle if done correctly. These animals show that genetics play a large part of our size. But reduced portions aren't always healthy. Elephants aren't supposes to be that skinny.

This is a reason that for some larger people I recommend that they eat more to lose weight. When the body gets all its nutrients, it operates well and weight loss is best achieved in a healthy environment. Your body needs the right tools to work. If a person is starving, the body is trying to maintain itself with reduced nutrients or a small toolbox. This situation can hinder all your efforts to lose weight.

In every case study I read about athletes with performance issues, the first and primary action is to make sure their getting their daily recommended intakes. Nutrition and portions must be balanced for healthy weight loss. That's particularly why I recommend unlimited fruits and vegetables. Below an outline of the Photo Shoot diet, you will have to tailor it to your personal preferences.

Photo Shoot Diet

If you're not sedentary and you already weight train and you only need to lose a little belly fat fast. This may help you get picture ready. This is not a permanent plan and should not be done more than a month. For larger clients I would recommend 2 days of weight training also. Also larger clients may not need to be as aggressive to lose the weight. Bigger people can lose weight faster with less work. Nice fact isn't it?

- First increase your vegetables. This will add nutrients and calories without adding fat.
- Increase your fiber. This will keep you full longer and reduce sugar in the blood, which will prevent fat storage.
- Increase your cardio by 3-5 hours weekly. You will burn more calories and aerobic leg movements are the best ab workout for reducing belly fat.
- Decrease animal products meat, dairy, fats, and oils. These are rich in fatty acids, which help in

making blood fat and fat storage.
■ Decrease alcohol. Alcohol is the fastest way to store fat. Consider it liquid fat.
■ Decrease overall calories. Use the Cup & Saucer. Eat your main meal at lunch. Make snacks veggies or fruit.
■ Decrease or cut all sugars. Sugar spikes insulin, which leads to fat storage. This especially includes decreasing artificial sweeteners to little or zero. (watch out for artificial sweeteners in carbs)
■ Lastly try to drink enough water to get you urine the color of light lemonade.

Fast weight loss is not the best strategy for long lasting results. So if you are a model, or have a special event coming here's your action plan. Remember 2 weeks is long enough for most people and no more than a month is still within reason. In the longer term use the Cup & Saucer plan.

Chapter 9

Eat with Your Hands

In June of 2010 the US government released its new eating guidelines using a plate to diagram the portions of each food groups to eat. I love it. It's easy to remember and follow. You look at it once and you have it forever. There's a lot of criticism about the protein portion of the plate since protein is a nutrient not a food.

Vegetables are protein sources also, a fact that's lost in the governments' diagram. Also the dairy portion seems to be a win for the food lobby. But overall it's great and lot better than the Food Pyramid.

Here's how you can make it better. The plate is not three-dimensional so how can you tell how much in ounces of the food to eat? Also if you're trying to lose weight, this is way too much food. Three big plates a day. Really this plate should be smaller, not like your normal dinner plate size. Considering the average meal is 800 to 1500 calories, this diagram my set some up for a diet failure.

To solve the dimension problem use the method mentioned earlier called, 'Eat With Your Hands.' Some nutritional guidelines give you options to remember like a deck of cards, two dice or a tennis ball. Here's an easier way to remember the amounts of each food categories. I call it, 'Eating with Your Hands' or 'Serving Sizes gets a Hand'. Here's the easier way to remember daily serving sizes. (Some nutritionist recommends more carbs and less fruits and veggies. That's good for maintaining weight not losing.)

Learn to eat with your hands. Here's how.

Make a fist
-This is the serving size for your rice, pasta, or potatoes

Open your Hand
-Here is the size for your meats

Two fingertips
-Serving size for cheese

Again make a fist
-Inside is your sauces, butters, and creams

Make two Fists
-These are your fruits and veggies

Cup one hand
-Here's your dessert. (Not required) you can trade this cupped hand for wine, beer, etc.

Dietary & Nutritional requirements can be easily met, with this simple method.

Chapter 10

How a Cup & Saucer Can Change Your Life.

This is the time when all the things we discussed earlier come together. The goal is to balance nutrition, portion control, cravings, and carb timing. I've gave much use to memory aids like. Pyramid Eating, R.A.P., Eat With Your Hands, Starting a Fire, the Fab Four, and Cup & Saucer. At this point, if you understand how all of these work I've done my job. If not, try again to learn these. They cover all the basics of weight loss nutrition you need to know.

For you this book has begun to grow handles and you're on the way to losing yours. Love handles that is.

The Cup & Saucer Meal Plan is the best example of Pyramid eating and it's your long-term strategy for health and weight loss. It puts heavy emphasis on natural real foods at the same time it can be tailored to individual cultural foods and taste. Every principle aforementioned can be incorporated in this way of eating. You may start by using the simplest form of the eating plan then as you gain experience make adaptations to bring it more in line with the principles you've learned.

There are three phases to the Cup & Saucer. Red, Yellow and Green.

Red: Stop the Madness

Modifying the timing of meals will help you to get control of your appetite, lose water weight and start using fat as fuel. You have to spend a day or two minimizing your breakfast and dinner sizes. Stop eating big meals at breakfast and dinner. Learn to eat real fruit and vegetables for snacks and change to a Pyramid eating style. Also spacing out your meals and snacks to about three hour intervals. For instance, breakfast at 8am, snack at 10:30 am, Lunch at 12 then another snack at 3pm, lastly diner at 6:00pm. Try not to eat much or anything at all within 3 hours of bed.

Yellow: Easy In

The Cup & Saucer emphasizes portion control, which is most people's biggest problem. It gets you the appropriate amount of calories for your body and goals. To lose weight I recommend you eat about 10 calories per pound. This is not a hard and fast rule because even the strictest of counters cannot accurately know how many calories they're consuming. Do not worry, that's why we have the cup and saucer.

Your breakfast should be the size of a teacup. Yes small. If you glance at serving sizes on cereal boxes the servings are not a full cup. Their 1/2 a cup or 2/3 cup size. Just use a teacup. Remember you can snack again before lunch but for now just put a little wood on the fire.

Lunchtime is on you. You know what to avoid. But your metabolism is likely up to speed now. Even if you put something not so good on the fire, you have the ability to burn it. If you have cravings this is the time to satisfy them. You don't have to live life without pizza or ice cream. Just be smart, if you're trying to lose weight make good choices but do eat and eat well at lunch. You have about 4-8 high metabolic hours to burn what you have eaten.

Dinner is slow and easy. Eat on a saucer, the one that comes with the teacup. Yes this is a very small plate; it's all you need before preparing to sleep. Your metabolism is slowing and there's no need for so much energy at this time.

Green: Keep Moving

The last stage helps you make appropriate choices in Protein, Carbs, and Fats. In the morning inside your saucer should be a good clean protein to help you stay full. Egg whites for example. Vegetables like spinach, mushrooms, tomatoes, onions or peppers will help you get the nutrients you need. Consider them multivitamins or diet pills. Use whole fiber to keep your blood sugar stable. If you can, drink coffee it's a stimulant. The energy will promote movement and thereby burn calories. At lunch learn to figuratively to 'Eat With Your Hands'. You must always find vegetables to eat with every meal. Here is where you may be most tempted to eat refined carbs. You can find good food if you are insistent. Don't fall into cutting back on lunch portions, you consistently need to and must eat here or you risk throwing your appetite and metabolism off the pattern you set. At Dinner time inside your saucer focus on clean, green, and lean foods. Whereas in the first phase of the Cup & Saucer you only focused on the portion, here you must also pay attention to content. Maybe a small salad along with your saucer will suit your taste.

Remember this is a 'Diet' in the original sense of the word; it's a way of life. You control and you tweak it to fit. It's a slow progressive way to eat better and consistently lose weight. You should not be hungry with the ability to eat so often. Unlimited fruits and vegetables are available. You can satisfy cravings daily if necessary. You don't need a diet because the way you're eating now will consistently move you in the right direction.

Again here's your 6 Meal Plan, fill it out with what you now know. Filling it out now will help your resolve and put it firmly in your memory.

Breakfast (small) where? home/restaurant
-protein source
-whole grain
-fruits
-vegetables

SNACK (fruit or veggie)

Lunch where? home/restaurant
-protein source
-whole grain
-fruits
-vegetables

SNACK (fruit or veggie)

Dinner (small) where? home/restaurant
-protein source
-whole grain
-fruits
-vegetables

Eat this way 5 days a week. Ideally you want more fruits & veggies
than anything else.

Breakfast (small) where? home/restaurant
-protein source
-whole grain
-fruits
-vegetables

SNACK (fruit or veggie)

Lunch where? home/restaurant
-protein source
-whole grain
-fruits
-vegetables

SNACK (fruit or veggie)

Dinner (small) where? home/restaurant
-protein source
-whole grain
-fruits
-vegetables

If you eat out, choose real whole lean meats, whole grains, and add every vegetable possible. Avoid if possible fried, & breaded foods.

Chapter 11

Bankruptcy, Carb Timing, & Calorie Deficits

So how do we use the entire product we stored over the years? Calorie Deficits and Metabolic Bankruptcy. It is at night when most of our bodies' repair and regrowth takes place. Just following Pyramid Eating particularly the Cup & Saucer will facilitate this. We want the body every night to set out unused stock. The only way is to use it up during the day.

Using too much can spark us to eat more so most fitness trainers will recommend only a 500-1000 calorie deficit a day. This is done best through a combination of diet and exercise. If possible an hour of moderate exercise daily can give you a deficit of 500 calories.

This is a hard sell for many people because if you had the motivation or opportunity to do this you would have it done already. So we will approach it this way, the more you lose the easier it will be to follow an exercise program. Start with 1 to 2 hours of exercise a week. This is a small moderate goal but we will maximize it with diet.

To create the Caloric Deficit or Metabolic Bankruptcy at the right time, focus on the evening meal. Breakfast as normal, moderate lunch, and light and early at dinner. Not going to bed hungry but not leaving anything for fat storage. For most people it going to be 300 calories or less at this time. You will have to work at this so see what's reasonable for you. Think long term. Eating nothing at night or in the morning isn't long term thinking. And if you find yourself in this pattern get help. It's neither normal nor healthy. Set a target, a bottom weight goal. Make that goal known to someone you trust. Consult your parent, trainer, nutritionist or doctor about the goal you set. When you reach the goal, you will have to work to break the pattern of weight loss. This seems like a good problem to have but be assured it can be a real problem. An underweight and a under nourished state can lead to death quicker than being overweight. If you find that you do not like the shape your body has taken, give it time to adjust as you weight train.

Remember you've lost fat and muscle and it takes time to find its balance and shape. Fat and muscle have hormones, so your body will have to work with a new hormonal composition. Remember perfection is not the goal; your view of perfection may well be a fantasy. The numbers you choose for your bottom weight will prevent you from going overboard. Be modest and realistic in setting this goal.

Chapter 12

Sweat The Big Stuff.

What's the reward for doing good? The opportunity and ability to do more. Likely you are similar to most of us, you fill your day in doing things for others. You like many people are a Giver, a busy one at that. In all your generosity you cannot afford any down time for yourself.

You would like to start an exercise program, because dieting alone is not enough. Exercising and eating well if only done in self-interest is not the most beneficial way to motivate yourself or anyone else. In fact answer this question, why are you too busy to exercise anyway?

The truth is that we all are Givers in varying degrees. Your giving is not a valid excuse. Why? Well, what is your best gift? You. Yes you want to give the best 'You' that you can give. Daily we prepare to give the best of ourselves that we can muster. Exercise and healthy eating is the same. It's helping you to continue to have the opportunities and ability to give the best possible 'you' for a long time. You are your best gift! Be aware that you can't do it all in any area. So our focus has to be on the most important of the lifestyle regimens for health and exercise and then progressively add to these. For now, make it your goal to focus on one of the principles listed below or just these four mwhen exercising or dieting.

The FITT principle is well known by virtually all exercise trainers. It helps us form a framework around a client's workout. You should know it and use it yourself for your diet as well as exercise.

Principle (F. I. T. T)

-FREQUENCY is how often you keep your diet & exercise protocols. Frequency is the most important protocol of all. Doing anything regularly will give some form of progress. What we do regularly is who we are. It defines us. Focus on frequency. Keep your exercise appointments even if their for just 15 minutes. Find a way to modify your exercise if something comes up that disrupts your schedule. The wonderful thing about some exercises is that they can be done anywhere in any clothing. For instance sitting leg lifts, triceps dips, toe raises, walking, ab work or lunges. Some may feel a little awkward doing triceps dips in the office. But we should not be embarrassed to do something in public beneficial for your health. If any embarrassment is called for it should be for not doing what benefits us. So, allow little to get in the way of using these as a strategy to keep your Frequency.

-INTENSITY of effort is usually a direct link to results. This is the second most important principle you have. Make it a goal to do a little more each time. Keep track of how fast and how hard you worked in previous workouts. Write it down and try to make incremental increases in your intensity.

-TIMING. Can you schedule 30 minutes each day for exercise? Every 3 hours you're encouraged to try small healthy foods with water. Why not make these times you involve yourself in some form moderate exercise before or after your meals or snacks. By the way, timing is just as important for what you consume in the way of foods. So remember the principles discussed in the previous chapter.

-TYPE building strength, endurance, or lean mass calls for different protocols. Heart health, weight loss/gain, strength or immune support requires a variety of dietary approaches. The saying, 'you are what you eat' and 'you are what you do' are true in these instances. Focus on exercises that raise and lower your heart rate. These will give you a better workout in less time.

Again of all these FREQUENCY is the most important. With good habits the others tend to fall in place. Regular exercise has so many benefits. There are even strong associations of exercise with reducing the effects of memory relates diseases.

The American Heart Association recommends 150 minutes of moderate exercise every week. This is said to reduce cancer risk, and diabetes.

American Journal of Clinical Nutrition 6/05, "weight training is effective in reducing the increased fat distribution around the waist that occurs in recovering anorexics... decreases rebound anorexia."

American Journal of Psychiatry 5/98 said, 'Exercise reduces panic attacks by half'

Group exercise 'boosts happiness'. Those doing group exercise feel happier than if they were on their own exercising alone. Exercising together appears to increase the level of the feel-good effect.

One Doctor a Emory University said if exercise was a pill it would be the most prescribed medicine in the world. It's that useful an available to everyone.

It's been reported that one elderly South African Golfer does 1000 sit-ups daily.

The take away for this book is that I want you to be productive in your efforts to lose weight and eat healthy. I've giving you overarching principles that you can apply to whatever diet or exercise regimens you desire. When you hear diet advice, use these principles to judge its effectiveness and practicality.

At this time, you have more knowledge of healthy than most basic exercise trainers. And you have a practical way of carrying it out. I expect those using these principles to lose weight, and make changes the same way negative effects in your diet came about, gradually and slowly, but safely. This is the long-term strategy not a cleanse or a fad. It's a way of life. You can ignore every new diet trend that comes your way.

There's no need to buy special foods, bars, programs, count calories or take pills. Save your money. You will lose weight, gradually and continually, the right way. Quick weight loss is not permanent weight loss. So many people gain all of the weight they lost back, even with the best of trainers. Personal Trainers long term success rate is only three percent. Things changed on the outside but nothing changed on the inside. The outside will always move to match the inside. You will be what you are on the inside. And you can change what you are, but only with good information and a realistic strategy to carry it out.

The Cup & Saucer is portion control, it's timing your meals effectively, it helps you to get the nutrients you need through real food, you do not go hungry with the Cup & Saucer and it allows rooms for your favorite foods. Lastly it's simple and easy to remember. That you can handle.

www.ingramcontent.com/pod-product-compliance
Lightning Source LLC
Chambersburg PA
CBHW060208290526
45789CB00003B/1205